MENOPAUSE REVIVAL POWER

HEALING YOUR BODYS HORMONAL SETTING WITH VIGOR

DISCLAIMER NOTICE:

Please note the information contained within the document is for educational and entertainment purposes only. All effort has been executed to present accurate, up to date, reliable, complete information. No warranties of any kind are declared or implied. Readers acknowledge that the author is not engaged in the rendering of legal, financial, medical or professional advice. The content within this book (Menopause Revival Power) has been derived from various sources. Please consult a licensed professional before attempting any techniques outlined in this book. By reading this document, the reader agrees that under no circumstances is the author responsible for any loses, direct or indirect, that are incurred because of the use of the information contained within this document, including but not limited to errors, omissions, or inaccuracies.

ISBN :9798332408748
written by: Reno Ben
year of publication: 2024

THIS BOOK BELONGS TO:

____

____

____

TABLE OF CONTENTS

Chapter 5:
Relationships Redefined
- 1. Partner Dynamics: Communicating Through Change
- 2. Family Matters: Bridging Generational Gaps
- 3. Friendship Fortresses: Strengthening Bonds

Chapter 6:
Sexual Renaissance
- 1. Intimacy After Menopause: Rekindling Passion
- 2. Body Positivity: Embracing Sensuality
- 3. Communication in the Bedroom: Honesty and Empathy

Chapter 7:
Health Beyond Menopause
- 1. Heart Health: Protecting Your Cardiovascular System
- 2. Bone Density: Strengthening Your Foundation
- 3. Cancer Awareness: Early Detection and Prevention

Chapter 8:
Stress less Living: Finding Balance Amidst Chaos
- 1. The Stress Epidemic: Understanding Its Impact on Menopause
- 2. Mindfulness Matters: Cultivating Calm in Daily Life
- 3. Stress-Busting Techniques: Strategies for Immediate Relief
- 4. Self-Care Rituals: Nurturing Your Well-being Amidst Responsibilities

Chapter 9:
Beauty Beyond Age: Embracing Your Radiance
- 1. Ageless Beauty: Rethinking Standards and Definitions
- 2. Skincare Secrets: Nourishing Your Skin Through Menopause
- 3. Makeup Mastery: Enhancing Your Features with Confidence
- 4. Hair Care Harmony: Embracing Changes with Grace

Chapter 10:

Confidence Redefined: Thriving in Your New Chapter

- 1. Inner Strength: Cultivating Confidence from Within
- 2. Body Love: Embracing and Celebrating Your Menopausal Body
- 3. Fashion Forward: Dressing for Success and Comfort
- 4. Power Poses and Presence: Projecting Confidence in Every Situation

INTRODUCTION

IINTRODUCTION:

Few events are as ubiquitous and unavoidable in the fabric of human existence as change. It's an all-pervasive force that molds our lives and drives us on a never-ending path of development, change, and self-discovery. And yet, in the clamor of life's ups and downs, there is one particular shift that shines as a light of opportunity as well as challenge: menopause.
With "Menopause Revival Power," we set out on a journey that goes beyond just accepting change; we plunge headfirst into the choppy seas of metamorphosis, driven by the steadfast conviction that every disruption harbors the potential for rebirth. Within the pages of this life-changing book, menopause is confronted not as a sign of decline but as a sacred threshold that calls us to let go of social expectations, accept the whole of who we are, and emerge renewed, invigorated, and completely unstoppable.

"Menopause Revival Power " is fundamentally an invitation to embrace the winds of change, dance to the beat of transition, and unlock the limitless potential that is dormant inside. By utilizing an extensive array of scientific studies, traditional knowledge, and firsthand accounts, [Author's Name] encourages readers to set out on a path of self-discovery and empowerment, where the turbulent phases of menopause are converted into a harmonious melody of opportunities.

But this is not just a book; it is a manifesto, a call to action for all women to take back control of their bodies, minds, and futures. We examine the widespread myths and misunderstandings about menopause through the prism of Menopause Revival Power," breaking the taboos of shame and silence that have long accompanied this holy journey. As a period when the masks of society expectations are discarded and the luminous essence of our actual selves is revealed, we celebrate menopause instead as a doorway to liberty.

We delve into the many aspects of this life-changing experience in "Menopause Revival Power," covering everything from the emotional landscape of identity redefinition to the physical expressions of hormonal imbalances. We negotiate the challenges of intimacy, sensuality, and self-image via open discussions and personal introspection, coming out on the other side with a renewed feeling of agency, honesty, and grace.

The fact that "Menopause Revival Power " reminds us that we are never alone on this journey of transition is possibly its most significant contribution to the community. We find comfort in the experiences that our sisters have shared inside these pages, and we gain strength from their tales, wisdom, and steadfast support.

Thus, my dear reader, know that you are not just turning the pages of a book when you set out on this life-changing journey— rather, you are embarking on a sacred pilgrimage to find, redefine, and celebrate the luminous essence of your new body. Accept the winds of change, for they carry with them the opportunity of endless possibilities, rejuvenation, and rebirth. Welcome to "Menopause Renewal Street," a place where change is honored as the spark that ignites our greatest evolutionary leap to date.

CHAPTER 1: UNVEILING MENOPAUSE

CHAPTER 1: Unveiling Menopause

Few events are as ubiquitous and unavoidable in the fabric of human existence as change. It's an all-pervasive force that molds our lives and drives us on a never-ending path of development, change, and self-discovery. And yet, in the clamor of life's ups and downs, there is one particular shift that shines as a light of opportunity as well as challenge: menopause.

With "Menopause Revival Power," we set out on a journey that goes beyond just accepting change; we plunge headfirst into the choppy seas of metamorphosis, driven by the steadfast conviction that every disruption harbors the potential for rebirth. Within the pages of this life-changing book, menopause is confronted not as a sign of decline but as a sacred threshold that calls us to let go of social expectations, accept the whole of who we are, and emerge renewed, invigorated, and completely unstoppable.

"The Menopause Revival Power is fundamentally an invitation to embrace the winds of change, dance to the beat of transition, and unlock the limitless potential that is dormant inside. By utilizing an extensive array of scientific studies, traditional knowledge, and firsthand accounts, [Author's Name] encourages readers to set out on a path of self-discovery and empowerment, where the turbulent phases of menopause are converted into a harmonious melody of opportunities.

But this is not just a book; it is a manifesto, a call to action for all women to take back control of their bodies, minds, and futures. We examine the widespread myths and misunderstandings about menopause through the prism of "Menopause Revival Power," breaking the taboos of shame and silence that have long accompanied this holy journey. As a period when the masks of society expectations are discarded and the luminous essence of our actual selves is revealed, we celebrate menopause instead as a doorway to liberty.

We delve into the many aspects of this life-changing experience in "Menopause Renewal Reset," covering everything from the emotional landscape of identity redefinition to the physical expressions of hormonal imbalances. We negotiate the challenges of intimacy, sensuality, and self-image via open discussions and personal introspection, coming out on the other side with a renewed feeling of agency, honesty, and grace.

The fact that "Menopause Revival Power" reminds us that we are never alone on this journey of transition is possibly its most significant contribution to the community. We find comfort in the experiences that our sisters have shared inside these pages, and we gain strength from their tales, wisdom, and steadfast support.

Thus, my dear reader, know that you are not just turning the pages of a book when you set out on this life-changing journey—rather, you are embarking on a sacred pilgrimage to find, redefine, and celebrate the luminous essence of your new body. Accept the winds of change, for they carry with them the opportunity of endless possibilities, rejuvenation, and rebirth. Welcome to "Menopause Revival Power," a place where change is honored as the spark that ignites our greatest evolutionary leap to date.

1. The Biological Shift: What's Happening Inside?

Menopause is a complicated symphony orchestrated by the slow loss of reproductive hormones, especially progesterone and estrogen. It is sometimes thought of as a biological necessity. Menstruation ends and menopause begins when women approach their late 40s to early 50s because their ovaries gradually produce fewer of these hormones. This biological shift involves a significant recalibrating of the body's hormonal landscape in addition to the cessation of monthly periods.

Menopause's biological symptoms differ from woman to woman, but frequent ones include mood swings, hot flashes, nocturnal sweats, dry vagina, and decreased libido. Even though they can be upsetting, these physical changes are a normal aspect of going through menopause and signify the body's shift into a new stage of life.

To handle the menopause with grace and empowerment, it is essential to comprehend its biological foundations. Women can embrace menopause as a life-changing journey of self-discovery and rejuvenation and develop a deeper respect for life's natural rhythms by deciphering the physiological changes taking place within their bodies.

2. Debunking Myths: Separating Fact from Fiction

Menopause has long been associated with myth and misinformation, which are reinforced by cultural stigmas and taboos. A culture of anxiety and uncertainty around this normal stage of life has been exacerbated by myths such as the idea that menopause marks the end of a woman's energy and that it invariably results in weight gain and libido loss.

Many of these myths are, in fact, just that—myths. Although menopause does cause physical changes, it does not mean that a woman's value or desirability is gone. Furthermore, weight gain and decreased libido are not always associated with menopause; rather, these changes are frequently impacted by a wide range of factors, such as lifestyle, genetics, and general health.

Through dispelling these misconceptions and distinguishing reality from fantasy, women may take back control of their menopausal journey and confidently and powerfully welcome this change. Equipped with precise information, individuals can confidently and clearly negotiate the menopausal transition, knowing that they are not going through this alone.

3. **Embracing the Transition: A New Phase of Womanhood**

Menopause is a time of life characterized by wisdom, resiliency, and inner strength, not the end of womanhood. It's a moment to honor the depth of our womanhood in all its complexity and to enjoy the wealth of experience that comes with growing older.

Menopause can be seen as a chance to let go of the limitations of youth and embrace the freedom that comes with age, rather than as a loss. Now is the perfect opportunity to rethink who we are and develop a closer bond with our bodies, minds, and spirits.

It takes bravery, vulnerability, and an openness to change to really accept the menopause. It necessitates that we let go of antiquated ideas of attractiveness and beauty in favor of accepting the beauty that results from self-acceptance and honesty. Women can regain their agency, voice, and power by accepting the menopause transition and coming out of it stronger, wiser, and more beautiful than before.

In summary, menopause is a complex process that includes emotional, psychological, and biological shifts. Women can traverse this transforming journey with grace, empowerment, and a renewed sense of purpose if they accept the transition as a new phase of femininity, understand the physiologic processes occurring within their bodies, and dispel the myths surrounding menopause. Welcome to "The New Body Menopause," a place where change is cherished as a means of bringing about personal growth and transformation rather than just accepted.

NOTE

CHAPTER 2:
NAVIGATING HORMONAL ROLLERCOASTER

NAVIGATING THE HORMONAL ROLLERCOASTER is the topic of Chapter Deux.

Menopause is frequently compared as riding a chaotic rollercoaster of hormonal changes, where each twist and turn brings new challenges and unexpected sensations. This is because menopause is characterized by a gradual shift in hormone levels. This chapter provides insights, methods, and powerful perspectives to help women traverse this transitional time with fortitude and grace. It conducts a deep dive into the physiological and emotional journey of menopause.

A Better Understanding of Hormonal Changes

A woman's hormonal landscape undergoes a dramatic change during menopause, which is defined by a steady drop in the production of estrogen and progesterone; this change is a big change. This variation in hormone levels causes a chain reaction of changes in both the body and the mind, including but not limited to hot flashes, nocturnal sweats, mood swings, and sleep difficulties.

The biological mechanisms that are responsible for these hormone fluctuations are investigated at the beginning of the chapter. The brain, pituitary gland, and ovaries are all important roles in the regulation of the menstrual cycle, and this article describes how diminishing hormone levels affect these parts of the body, as well as the broader consequences for overall health and well-being.

Acceptance of Your Physical Changes

One of the most important aspects of successfully navigating the hormonal rollercoaster that is menopause is to acknowledge and comprehend the bodily changes that accompany this period of growth. Some of the frequent symptoms that are discussed in this chapter include vaginal dryness, weight gain, and changes in the texture of the skin and hair. The chapter also provides guidance on how to manage these changes through the use of self-care practices, such as nutrition and exercise.

Additionally, it emphasizes the significance of maintaining frequent health tests and meetings with healthcare specialists in order to keep track of bone health, cardiovascular risk factors, and other potential health issues that may manifest themselves during menopause for women.

The Management of Emotional Shifts and Changes

It is not just a period of physical transition, but also a period of emotional re-calibration that occurs throughout menopause. The psychological components of menopause are discussed in this chapter. These features include mood swings, impatience, and anxiety, all of which can be made worse by hormonal abnormalities.

This article explores useful coping tactics, such as mindfulness techniques, stress management, and cognitive behavioral therapy (CBT), with the goal of navigating emotional changes with resilience and self-awareness. In addition to this, it highlights the significance of social support networks, peer groups, and counseling services in terms of offering emotional validation and solidarity during this period of transition.

Coping Strategies and Support

Navigating the hormonal rollercoaster of menopause requires adaptive coping strategies and a supportive network. This chapter explores various approaches to managing menopausal symptoms and promoting well-being during this transformative phase:

Lifestyle Modifications:
Adopting a healthy diet, regular exercise, and adequate sleep can help alleviate symptoms and promote overall health.

Hormone Replacement Therapy (HRT):
Discussing the pros and cons of HRT with healthcare providers can help women make informed decisions about managing severe symptoms.

Mind-Body Techniques:
Practices such as yoga, meditation, and deep breathing exercises can reduce stress, improve sleep, and enhance emotional resilience.

Support Networks:
Connecting with peers, support groups, or healthcare professionals who specialize in menopause can provide validation, information, and emotional support.

Improvements to the Quality of Life

The chapter urges women to prioritize their quality of life and well-being within the context of the hormonal rollercoaster that they are experiencing. The article explores holistic approaches to the management of menopausal symptoms, which include alternative therapies such as acupuncture, herbal supplements, and adaptations to lifestyle such as yoga and meditation.

In addition, the chapter examines the effects that menopause has on intimate relationships and the quality of those relationships, providing advice on how to communicate, preserve sexual health, and keep an emotional connection with partners.

Education with the Goal of Empowerment

At the heart of successfully managing the hormonal rollercoaster that is menopause is the empowerment that comes from acquiring information and understanding. This chapter offers women with evidence-based information on hormone replacement therapy (HRT), including its advantages, dangers, and alternatives. This information empowers women to make informed decisions about their health in cooperation with healthcare providers.

Additionally, it promotes proactive self-advocacy in healthcare settings, with the goal of arguing for tailored treatment regimens that are in accordance with the preferences and values of the entire individual.

Recognizing Menopause as a Process of Personal Growth and Development

It is ultimately about embracing this transforming journey with perseverance, self-compassion, and a sense of strength in order to successfully navigate the hormonal rollercoaster that is menopause. The chapter comes to a close with a collection of uplifting accounts of women who have embraced menopause as a period of regeneration, growth, and self-discovery. These accounts provide readers who are beginning their own menopausal journey with hope and encouragement.

This chapter provides women with the knowledge and tools necessary to negotiate the rollercoaster ride of menopause with grace and vigor. It does this by providing a detailed analysis of the hormonal changes, physical symptoms, emotional obstacles, and empowerment methods that are connected with menopause.

NOTE

CHAPTER 3: REINVENTING WELLNESS: LIFESTYLE CHANGES FOR MENOPAUSAL WOMEN

Changes in lifestyle advice for menopausal women are discussed in Chapter 3, "Reinventing Wellness."

As a woman goes through menopause, she undergoes a significant change in her life, which necessitates a reassessment of her health priorities and the lifestyle choices she makes. This chapter examines how women can empower themselves to manage menopause with vitality and resilience by acknowledging the importance of wellbeing and making focused changes to their lifestyle.

Taking a Holistic Approach to Wellness

The menopause is not merely a biological process; rather, it is a journey of transformation that covers not only the physical but also the emotional and spiritual aspects of healthcare. In order to improve one's overall quality of life during this period of transition, it is important to embrace holistic wellness, which entails treating all elements of well-being with care.

Techniques for Maintaining Hormonal Balance Through Diet

In the management of menopausal symptoms and in the maintenance of overall health, nutrition is an extremely important factor. In this section, we will discuss dietary options that can help reduce symptoms, maintain hormonal balance, and support long-term wellness:

- Nutritional Balance: Putting an emphasis on a diet that is abundant in fruits, vegetables, whole grains, and lean proteins can offer important nutrients and maintain hormonal homeostasis.

Phytoestrogens: Consuming foods that are high in phytoestrogens, such as soy products, flaxseeds, and legumes, may be able to alleviate hot flashes and other symptoms that are connected with a decrease in estrogen levels.

- Omega-3 Fatty Acids: Consuming foods that are rich in omega-3 fatty acids, such as walnuts, flaxseed oil, and fatty fish, can be beneficial to the health of the heart, as well as to cognitive function and mood stability.

In order to better control hot flashes, sleep difficulties, and mood swings, it is helpful to limit the consumption of foods that are known to be triggers. These foods include coffee, alcohol, spicy meals, and refined carbohydrates.

Strength training and resilience training exercises

During menopause, it is essential to engage in regular physical activity in order to preserve bone density, muscle strength, cardiovascular health, and mental well-being. This part of the article discusses the advantages of physical activity and offers suggestions for incorporating physical activity into daily activities, including the following:

- Aerobic Exercise: Participating in activities such as brisk walking, swimming, or cycling can enhance cardiovascular fitness, promote weight control, and boost mood. Other forms of aerobic exercise include swimming and cycling.

Incorporating resistance exercises using weights or resistance bands into your workout routine is an effective way to maintain muscle mass, improve bone density, and support joint health thanks to strength training.

It is possible to enhance flexibility and balance by engaging in activities such as yoga, tai chi, or stretching exercises. These activities also help to lower the risk of falling.

Techniques for Mind-Body Integration and Stress Management

It is possible for menopause to be accompanied by elevated levels of stress, which can have an effect on the quality of sleep, the stability of mood, and overall well-being. In this section, we will discuss practical tactics for managing stress as well as mind-body approaches that promote relaxation, resilience, and emotional equilibrium:

- **Meditation focused on mindfulness:** Through the practice of mindfulness practices, one can reduce stress, improve their ability to regulate their emotions, and boost their general mental clarity.

Exercising your deep breathing may include: Inducing relaxation responses, lowering anxiety, and improving the quality of sleep can be accomplished by the utilization of either deep breathing exercises or progressive muscle relaxation techniques.

Treatments that involve biofeedback and relaxation techniques: Monitoring and managing stress responses can be accomplished by the utilization of biofeedback devices or relaxation therapy, which in turn promotes both physiological and psychological well-being.

Proper sleeping hygiene and rejuvenating sleep

A good night's sleep is necessary for maintaining hormonal equilibrium, maintaining cognitive function, and maintaining overall health during menopause. In the following part, we will explore many tactics and practices for improving restorative sleep, including sleep hygiene:

In order to establish a regular pattern of sleep: Developing a regular sleep pattern and routine for going to bed sends a message to the body that it is time to relax, which in turn improves the quality and duration of sleep.

- "Optimizing Sleep Environment" refers to the process of creating a comfortable and conducive surroundings for sleeping, which includes the use of appropriate bedding, the regulation of temperature, and the reduction of light and noise disturbances.

Reduce your exposure to blue light and promote natural circadian rhythms that are beneficial to sleep by limiting the amount of time you spend in front of electronic devices before going to bed.

Adopting a Wellness Approach to Menopause

Women are able to handle the transition from menopause to postmenopause with a sense of strength and vigor if they embrace holistic wellness and make focused changes to their lifestyle. The objective of this chapter is to equip women with actionable techniques that will enable them to maximize their health, improve their resilience, and embrace a revitalized sense of well-being at this period of their lives that is very transforming.

NOTE

CHAPTER 4: EMPOWERING YOUR MIND: MENTAL HEALTH AND COGNITIVE VITALITY

Chapter 4: Empower Your Mind: Mental Health and Cognitive Vitality

This chapter of "Menopause Revival Power" delves deeply into the mind, creating a sanctuary where resilience, empowerment, and transformation coexist with the violent waves of hormonal transition.

1. The Emotional Journey of Menopause

Menopause is an emotional symphony, a kaleidoscope of feelings that ebb and flow with hormonal variations. During this transitional stage of life, women travel a maze of emotional landscapes, from the highs of newly discovered freedom to the lows of existential pondering.

It is critical to grasp that these feelings are not transitory moments, but rather strong messages that reveal the depths of our deepest aspirations and concerns. By embracing and acknowledging these emotions, women can begin on a path of self-discovery, gaining a better understanding of themselves and their needs.

2. Maintaining Cognitive Brilliance

As menopause progresses, there are subtle variations in cognitive function—a dance of memory lapses, mental fog, and periods of clarity. While these changes may be concerning, they are not symptomatic of cognitive deterioration, but rather reflect the complex interplay of hormones, stress, and age.

To maintain cognitive vibrancy during menopause, engage in mind nourishing activities such as puzzles, conversations that pique curiosity, and moments of seclusion that encourage contemplation. Women can continue to develop intellectually by challenging and nourishing their brains.

3. Empower Your Mind: Strategies for Resilience

Empowering your mind during menopause is a process that includes self-compassion, self-awareness, and self-empowerment. It starts with recognizing the intricacies of the menopausal experience and accepting the entire range of emotions that come with it.

Practicing mindfulness and meditation can help women find inner calm in the midst of hormonal upheaval, while seeking help from mental health specialists or support groups can give a safe space for processing emotions and gaining perspective.

Furthermore, prioritizing self-care—such as regular exercise, nutritious eating, and enough sleep—can promote both emotional and physical well-being, building the groundwork for resilience and empowerment during menopause.

Finally, empowering your mind during menopause is a voyage of self-discovery that encourages women to reach their full emotional and cognitive potential. Women can manage this transitional stage of life with grace, resilience, and a newfound sense of strength if they acknowledge the nuances of the menopausal experience, cultivate resilience, and embrace the power of self-care. Welcome to "Menopause Renewal Reset," where mental wellness and cognitive vigor are more than simply goals, but guiding principles on the journey to self-discovery and empowerment.

NOTE

CHAPTER 5:
RELATIONSHIPS
REDEFINED

Chapter 5: Relationships redefined

The physical and mental changes that a woman goes through during menopause are frequently used to frame the transition. However, what is generally ignored is the enormous impact that this stage may have on relationships. As you go through menopause, your relationships with your partner, family, friends, and, most importantly, with yourself are in change. This chapter investigates how menopause alters these relationships and provides advice on how to navigate this transition with grace, understanding, and empowerment.

1.Changing Dynamics with Your Partner.
 Emotional intimacy
Menopause can cause dramatic shifts in emotional intimacy with your partner. Hormonal variations can cause mood swings, anger, and worry, straining even the most stable relationships. However, it also provides an opportunity to strengthen emotional ties. Open and honest discussion about your experiences might help your spouse have a better understanding and empathy.

Strategies to Improve Emotional Intimacy:
1. Open Communication: Talk about your emotions, anxieties, and expectations with your partner. Share information on menopause and how it impacts you.

2. Emotional Support: Seek and offer emotional support. Engage in activities that foster emotional intimacy, such as date evenings, common hobbies, or simply spending quality time together.
3. Therapy and Counseling: Couples therapy can help you manage the emotional ups and downs. A professional can help you improve your relationship during this time.

Physical intimacy

Menopause can also have an impact on the physical aspects of relationships. Vaginal dryness, decreased libido, and intercourse discomfort are all frequent but tolerable symptoms. The goal is to tackle these challenges with care and a readiness to adapt and try new methods of preserving physical connection.

Maintaining Physical Intimacy:

1. Medical Interventions: Ask your doctor about treatments for vaginal dryness and other physical problems. Lubricants, moisturizers, and hormone therapy can have a considerable impact.

2. Experimentation: Look into new ways to connect physically. This can involve nonsexual touch, massage, or simply being physically close.

3. Open dialogue: Communicate openly with your partner about your physical demands and restrictions. Mutual understanding and patience are critical.

Developing Family Relationships

Children.

For many mothers, menopause coincides with their children reaching adulthood and becoming self-sufficient. This change can elicit a range of emotions, including feelings of loss and newfound freedom. It's time to reinvent your role as a parent and try new ways to connect with your children.

How to Navigate Changes With Children:

1. Letting Go: Accept and value your children's independence. Believe in their abilities to manage their own life.

2. New Bonds: Encourage a new type of relationship built on mutual respect and adult-to-adult engagement. Discover shared interests and activities to enjoy together.

3. help and Guidance: While taking a step back, continue to be a source of wisdom and help for others.

Aging Parents

As you traverse menopause, you may simultaneously be caring for aging parents. This dual duty of caretaker can be difficult but also extremely rewarding. Balancing your demands with those of your parents necessitates careful consideration and assistance.

Balanced Caregiving:
1. Seek Support: Don't be afraid to seek for assistance from siblings, other family members, or professional caretakers.
2. Self-Care: Put your health and well-being first. Remember, you cannot pour from an empty cup.
3. Communication: Maintain open channels of communication with your parents. Understand their requirements and preferences, and include them in decision-making.

Friendships Transformed
Deepening Connections
Friendships frequently take on new meaning throughout menopause. Friends can offer empathy, share their experiences, and serve as a support system. This stage provides an opportunity to strengthen existing friendships and make new, significant connections.

Creating Supportive Friendships:
1. Honesty and Vulnerability: Discuss your experiences and feelings with close friends. Vulnerability can help strengthen friendships.
2. Support Groups: Join or create menopause support groups. Sharing with people who are going through similar circumstances can be really validating.
3. Social Activities: Participate in activities that provide enjoyment and company. Discover what brings you together, whether it's a reading club, a hiking group, or an art class.

Reassessing Toxic Relationships.

Menopause is also an opportunity to reconsider relationships that no longer serve you. Emotional well-being is critical, and you may need to detach yourself from toxic relationships that deplete your energy and happiness.

Manage Toxic Relationships:
1. Establish Boundaries: Clearly establish and explain your boundaries. Protect your emotional space.
2. Limit Interaction: Spend less time with people that constantly bring negativity into your life.
3. Seek Closure: When required, seek closure in your relationship. Sometimes letting go is the healthiest option.

 The Relationship With Yourself

Self-discovery and Acceptance

Menopause is an intense era of self-discovery. Your identity evolves alongside your physical form. Embracing these changes with self-compassion and curiosity can help you get a better understanding and acceptance of yourself.

Embracing Self-Discovery:
1. Self-Reflection: Allow time for contemplation. Journaling, meditation, and therapy can all aid in self-discovery.
2. appreciate Milestones: Recognize and appreciate your accomplishments and milestones, large and little.
3. Self-Love: Develop your self-love and acceptance. Affirm your worth and beauty, despite of society expectations.

Health and Wellness.

Prioritizing health and wellness is critical during menopause. This is the moment to prioritize your physical, mental, and spiritual well-being. Prioritizing wellness:
1. Healthy Lifestyle: Eat a well-balanced diet, exercise regularly, and get plenty of sleep. These are essential for your general well-being.
2. Mind-Body Practices: Use yoga, tai chi, or mindfulness meditation to connect with your body and alleviate stress.
3. Medical Care: Stay current on your health. Regular check-ups and following medical recommendations are vital.

Rediscovering Passions

Menopause can be a time to rediscover and pursue loves and interests that were put on hold earlier in life.

Pursuing Passions:
1. interests and Interests: Revitalize old or discover new interests. Find something that excites you, whether it's painting, gardening, or learning a new language.
2. Volunteering: Participate in voluntary activities. Giving back to the community may be quite fulfilling.
3. Continued Learning: Sign up for courses or classes. Lifelong learning keeps the mind active and provides new opportunities for growth and fulfillment.

conclusion:

Menopause is a transitional stage that alters relationships on multiple levels. It's a period of transition, but also one of opportunity. You may negotiate these transitions with resilience and grace by embracing open communication, seeking help, and putting self-discovery and wellness first. Remember that this journey is about rediscovering yourself as well as changing your connections with others. Celebrate this new phase, and let it serve as a reminder of your resilience, adaptability, and unwavering capacity for love and connection.

NOTE

CHAPTER 6:
SEXUAL RENAISSANCE

Chapter 6: Sexual Renaissance.

Menopause signifies the end of a woman's reproductive years, but it does not signal the end of her sexual life. In fact, this change may signal a "Sexual Renaissance," a period of renewed sexual exploration, intimacy, and satisfaction. This chapter digs into how menopause might change your sexual life, discussing both the obstacles and opportunities that come with this new stage.

Understanding the Changes.

 Physical Changes

Menopause causes considerable hormonal alterations, specifically a decrease in estrogen and progesterone. These changes can affect your body in a variety of ways, including sexual health and function.

Key physical changes:
1. Vaginal Dryness and Atrophy: Low estrogen levels can cause thinning and dryness of the vaginal walls, resulting in discomfort during intercourse.
2. Lowered Libido: Hormonal variations may reduce sexual desire.
3. Changes in Sexual Response: Changes in blood flow and sensitivity might impact arousal and orgasm.

Managing Physical Change:
1. Lubricants and Moisturizers: Over-the-counter treatments can help relieve dryness and irritation.
2. Hormone Therapy: Ask your doctor about estrogen or other hormone treatments that can help with physical symptoms.
3. Regular Sexual Activity: Regular sexual activity helps enhance blood flow and keep your vagina healthy.

Emotional and Psychological Changes

Menopause can have an emotional and psychological impact on your sexual life as well. Mood swings, anxiety, and body image changes can all impact sexual desire and fulfillment.

How to Navigate Emotional Changes:
1. Mindfulness and Meditation: Techniques that relieve stress and promote emotional well-being can improve your sexual experience.
2. Therapy and Counseling: Talking to a therapist can assist with anxiety, despair, and body image concerns.
3. Open Communication: Talk about your feelings with your partner to improve understanding and closeness.

Rediscovering Desire

Reframe Sexuality

Menopause provides an opportunity to redefine your sexuality. With reproductive worries resolved, you may concentrate on pleasure and connection without the stress of fertility.

Embracing a New Perspective:
1. Focus on Pleasure: Move the attention away from performance and outcomes and toward enjoyment of the event.
2. Explore Fantasies: Allow yourself to experience sexual fantasies and desires that you may have previously suppressed.
3. Redefine Intimacy: Intimacy is more than just intercourse. Investigate alternative types of connection, including sensuous touch, massage, and non-sexual affection.

Improving Sexual Wellness

Improving your entire sexual well-being can revitalize your sex experience and boost satisfaction.

To increase sexual wellness, consider strengthening the pelvic floor muscles.

2. Healthy Lifestyle: A well-balanced diet, frequent exercise, and appropriate sleep all help to improve overall health and sexual health.

3. Sexual Health Check-Ups: Schedule regular visits with your healthcare physician to address any physical issues affecting your sexual health.

Reconnect with Your Partner

Communication and Connection.

Open and honest conversation with your partner is essential at this time. Discussing your needs, anxieties, and desires can lead to a more meaningful sexual connection.

Strategies for Effective Communication:

1. Scheduled Conversations: Set aside time to discuss your sexual connection without interruptions.

2. Use "I" Statements: Express your own feelings and needs instead of criticizing or blaming your partner.

3. Listen Actively: Show empathy and avoid passing judgment on your partner's problems and goals.

Experiment and Exploration

Menopause might be an opportunity to explore new aspects of your sexual relationship. Experimenting with various hobbies and techniques can provide freshness and excitement.

thoughts for Exploration

1. Erotic reading and Films: Sharing erotic reading or films might inspire new thoughts and imaginations.

2. Sex Toys and Accessories: Adding sex toys can provide diversity and pleasure.

3. Role-Playing and Fantasy: Engaging in role-playing or discussing fantasies can rekindle desire and intimacy.

Accepting Self-Pleasure

Self-pleasure, often known as masturbation, remains an important element of sexual health and wellness following menopause. It's an opportunity to explore your own body and discover what makes you happy.

Benefits of Self-Pleasure:
1. Increased Awareness: Understanding your own sexual responses might help you have better sex with your partner.
2. Reduced Stress: Masturbation causes the release of endorphins, which can help with stress reduction and mood improvement.
3. Enhanced Sexual Confidence: Understanding what you appreciate might boost your confidence in sexual interactions.

Self-exploration

Use this opportunity to rediscover your body and find new methods to enjoy pleasure.
Tips for Self-Exploration:
1. Mindful Masturbation: Concentrate on the feelings and emotions of the encounter rather than racing into climax.
2. Varied Techniques: Experiment with various techniques, speeds, and pressures to see what feels best.
3. Erotic Aids: Use lubricants, vibrators, or other toys to improve your experience.

Navigating Challenges

Managing Pain and Discomfort

Pain and discomfort during sex can be serious issues during menopause, but it's vital to remember that there are remedies.

Dealing With Pain:
1. Consult a Specialist: A healthcare specialist who specializes in sexual health can provide treatment and advise.
2. Gradual Introduction: If penetration is uncomfortable, begin with non-penetrative activities before progressively reintroducing penetration.
3. Use Lubricants*: Using lubricants liberally can help to alleviate dryness and friction.

Coping with Lowered Libido

A drop in libido is common throughout menopause, but it does not have to limit your sexual happiness.
Increasing Libido:
1. Hormonal Treatments: Discuss hormone replacement therapy with your doctor.
2. Aphrodisiacs and Supplements: Some women find natural aphrodisiacs or supplements beneficial, but you should discuss with your doctor first.
3. Focused Intimacy: Do activities that promote emotional and physical intimacy without the strain of intercourse.

Accepting a New Sexual Identity

Redefining Beauty and Sensuality.
Menopause provides an opportunity to reassess what beauty and sensuality mean to you. This stage of life can be powerful, providing a revitalized sense of self-esteem and attractiveness.

Embracing New Definitions:
1. Celebrate Your Body: Value your body's strength and resilience. Concentrate on the areas of your body that give you pleasure and satisfaction.
2. Confidence-Building things: Try things that make you feel confident and beautiful, such as dance, yoga, or fashion.
3. Positive Affirmations: Use positive affirmations to help you maintain a healthy and empowering self-image.

Community and Connection.

Finding a network of women who are going through menopause can offer support, validation, and shared experiences.

Establishing Community:
1. Support Groups: Join a menopause support group online or in your community.
2. Workshops and Seminars: Participate in workshops and seminars about sexual health and wellness throughout menopause.
3. Social Networks: Connect with friends who are going through similar circumstances and offer advise and support.

Conclusion:

Menopause does not mean the end of your sexual life; rather, it might mark the beginning of a sexual renaissance. Understanding and treating physical and mental changes, exploring new dimensions of intimacy, and embracing self-discovery can help you turn this phase into one of increased sexual energy and delight. This journey is about reclaiming your sexual health and discovering new ways to feel pleasure and connect. Celebrate this period of transition and embrace the potential of your sexual renaissance.

NOTE

CHAPTER 7:
HEALTH BEYOND
MENOPAUSE

Chapter 7: Health Beyond Menopause.

When you reach menopause, you begin a new stage of life that can be as enriching and fulfilling as any other. The post-menopausal years, also known as the "third age," provide distinct opportunities and challenges. Beyond menopause, health is about more than just controlling symptoms; it's about embracing holistic wellness, finding balance, and thriving.

Accepting a New Chapter

Menopause signals the end of menstruation and reproductive years, yet it does not mean the end of vitality and growth. Many women find that this interval allows them to rediscover their personal objectives, relationships, and self-care. With extended life spans, the postmenopausal years can last several decades, making it critical to emphasize health and well-being.

Understanding the Changes

Post-menopause causes physiological changes that can affect many aspects of health:

1. Hormonal Shifts: Following menopause, estrogen levels fall considerably. This hormonal shift has the potential to influence bone density, cardiovascular health, and skin suppleness.
2. Bone Health: A decrease in estrogen can cause osteoporosis, which makes bones more weak and susceptible to fractures.
3. Cardiovascular Health: Estrogen protects the heart. Lower amounts may raise the risk of heart disease.
4. Metabolism: Metabolism frequently slows, resulting in probable weight gain and body composition alterations.

Understanding these changes allows you to make more educated decisions about health management. Regular check-ups with healthcare practitioners are required to monitor these elements and implement preventive measures.

Holistic Approaches to Well-Being

A comprehensive approach to health after menopause entails addressing physical, mental, and emotional well-being. Here are some crucial methods to consider:

1. Nutrition: -Balanced Diet: Consume fruits, vegetables, whole grains, lean meats, and healthy fats. Foods high in calcium and vitamin D are especially beneficial for bone health.
   - Hydration: Drinking enough water helps maintain skin suppleness, assists digestion, and promotes overall bodily processes.
   - Supplies: Consult your healthcare professional about the need for supplements, particularly calcium, vitamin D, and omega-3 fatty acids.

2. Physical Activity: - Strength Training: Increases muscular mass, bone density, and metabolic rate.
   - Cardiovascular Exercise: Walking, swimming, and cycling boost heart health and stamina.
   - Flexibility and Balance: Yoga and Pilates improve your flexibility, balance, and mental clarity.

3. Mental Health: - Mindfulness and Meditation: These activities can reduce stress, improve emotional regulation, and boost general mental well-being.
   • Cognitive Health: Engage in brain-stimulating activities like puzzles, reading, and acquiring new skills.

4. Sleep Hygiene: - Consistent Routine: Stick to a regular sleep schedule to promote restorative sleep.
   - Sleep Environment: Create a peaceful sleeping environment with little light and noise.
   - Mindful Practices: Deep breathing and progressive muscle relaxation might improve sleep.

Preventive Healthcare

Preventive health care becomes even as important after menopause. Regular screenings and check-ups can spot any concerns early on, improving outcomes:

1. Bone Density Tests: Regular bone density tests help to monitor bone health and prevent osteoporosis.
2. Cardiovascular Screening: Regular examinations for blood pressure, cholesterol, and heart function can help avoid heart disease.
3. Cancer Screenings: Maintain routine screenings for breast, cervical, and colorectal cancer.
4. Eye and Dental Health: Regular eye exams and dental check-ups are required because changes in eyesight and oral health are normal with age.

Embracing Change with a Positive Mindset

A happy outlook can have a substantial impact on health results. Accepting this new phase with hope and an open mind can result in a more fulfilled existence. Here are some techniques to promote positivity:

1. Community and Connection: Stay in touch with friends and family. Participate in social events and join support groups to share your experiences and receive assistance.

2. Purpose and Passion: Engage in things that bring you joy and a sense of purpose, such as hobbies, volunteering, or exploring new interests.

3. Self-compassion: Be kind to oneself. Recognize and embrace the changes that your body undergoes, and concentrate on what you can do to preserve and improve your health.

The Journey Forward

The journey beyond menopause provides an opportunity to rethink what health and well-being mean to you. You may confidently and vitally handle this phase by embracing holistic techniques, preventive care, and a good outlook. This stage of life, characterized by wisdom and experience, has the possibility for further development, discovery, and fulfillment.

NOTE

CHAPTER 8:
STRESS LESS LIVING: FINDING BALANCE AMIDST CHAOS

Chapter 8: Stress Less Living: Finding Balance Among Chaos

Stress appears to be an unavoidable companion in today's fast-paced world. Finding equilibrium in the midst of chaos is critical for postmenopausal women's general well-being. This chapter delves into ways for stress management, resilience building, and living a harmonious life despite external constraints.

Understanding Stress in the Postmenopausal Phase

Stress is the body's reaction to any demand or threat, and it might appear physically, emotionally, or psychologically. During and after menopause, the body experiences major hormonal changes that might enhance stress responses. Common stressors at this stage of life include:

1. Physical Changes include weight fluctuations, sleep problems, and other menopausal symptoms.
2. Emotional Shifts: Mood swings, worry, and feelings of loss or bewilderment as you enter this new chapter of life.
3. External Pressures: Job commitments, caregiving responsibilities for elderly parents or grandchildren, and societal expectations.

Understanding these pressures is the first step towards their successful management. Recognizing that stress is a normal aspect of life enables us to tackle it with techniques for lessening its impact and promoting a balanced lifestyle.

The Effects of Chronic Stress

Chronic stress can have negative impacts on health, particularly in postmenopausal women.
1. Cardiovascular Health: Chronic stress raises the risk of hypertension, heart disease, and a stroke.

2. Mental Health: Chronic stress can cause anxiety, depression, and cognitive impairment.

3. Immune System: Stress impairs the immune system, leaving the body more vulnerable to sickness.

4. Digestive System: Stress can worsen digestive problems including IBS and acid reflux.

Given these potential consequences, it is critical to use stress-reduction tactics and lifestyle modifications that promote a more balanced and healthy life.

Strategies for Stress-Free Living

1. Mindfulness and Meditation: - Mindfulness Practices: Practice staying present in the moment. Deep breathing, body scanning, and mindful eating are all effective stress-reduction techniques.

   - Meditation: Regular meditation helps to relax the mind, reduce anxiety, and increase general mental clarity. Even a few minutes each day can make a difference.

2. Physical exercise: - Regular Exercise: Physical exercise produces endorphins, a natural mood enhancer. Include activities that you enjoy, such as walking, yoga, swimming, and dancing.

   - Mind-Body Exercises: Practices such as yoga and tai chi mix physical activity with mental attention, lowering stress and increasing general health.

3. Healthy Lifestyle Choices: - Nutrition: Consume a balanced diet with fruits, vegetables, whole grains, and lean protein. Avoid caffeine and sugar, as they might cause stress.

   - Sleep hygiene: Prioritize sleep by sticking to a regular sleep schedule, providing a relaxing environment, and avoiding electronics before bed.

4. Emotional Well-Being: - Journaling: Writing down your thoughts and feelings can aid in emotional processing and stress reduction.

   - Therapy and Counselling: Professional help can provide skills for stress management and resolving underlying problems.

   - Social Connections: Maintain close relationships with friends and family. Social support is an important stress-reduction mechanism.

5. Time Management and Organization: - Prioritize Tasks: Prioritize the most critical tasks and delegate or eliminate unnecessary ones.

   - Create Realistic Goals: Break down activities into smaller chunks and appreciate little accomplishments.

   - Create a Routine: Creating a daily routine helps provide structure and lessen the chaos that causes stress.

6. Hobbies and Recreation: - Participate in Activities You Enjoy: Hobbies offer a creative outlet and a reprieve from daily stresses. Find enjoyable pastimes, such as painting, gardening, reading, or playing an instrument.

   - Travel and Exploration: If feasible, discover new locations and experiences. Travel can provide a new perspective and a much-needed reprieve from daily stress.

Building Resilience

Resilience is the ability to adapt to and recover from stressors. Building resilience entails:

1. Positive Thinking: Develop a positive mindset by focusing on appreciation and the wonderful things in your life. Reframe difficulties as chances for advancement.
2. Self-Compassion: Show oneself kindness and understanding, especially during difficult times.
3. Adaptability: Approach life's problems with an open mind and a flexible attitude.

Creating a Harmonious Environment

Your environment might have a major impact on your stress levels. Consider the following.

1. Declutter and Organize: A clean environment can provide a sense of peace and control.
2. Nature and the Outdoors: Spend time in nature. Studies have shown that natural environments can reduce stress and boost happiness.
3. Personal Sanctuary: Create an area in your home where you may unwind and recover. This could be a comfortable reading nook, a meditation area, or a tranquil garden.

Conclusion: Thriving Among Chaos

Stress is an inherent part of life, but it does not have to consume your post-menopausal years. By taking a holistic approach to stress management, you may find balance and thrive in the midst of chaos. Embrace mindfulness, prioritize self-care, and develop resilience to help you manage this phase with grace and power. Remember that the goal is not to completely remove stress, but to manage it in a way that improves your general well-being and allows you to live a satisfying, harmonious life.

NOTE

CHAPTER 9:
BEAUTY BEYOND AGE: EMBRACING YOUR RADIANCE

Chapter 9: Beauty Beyond Age: Embracing Your Radiance

Beauty is a timeless and nuanced idea that defies age. As you progress through the postmenopausal years, appreciating your individual brilliance becomes an uplifting journey of self-discovery and acceptance. This chapter delves into how to enjoy your beauty at any age, offering practical advice and insights on cultivating your inner and outer glow.

Redefining Beauty

Society frequently associates beauty with youth, yet true beauty is timeless. It includes confidence, integrity, and wisdom gained over a lifetime. Post menopause is an opportunity to redefine beauty on your own terms, concentrating on what makes you feel energetic and alive.

Inner Radiance: Developing Confidence and Self-Love.

1. Self-Acceptance: - Embrace Change. Accept the normal changes that your body experiences. Celebrate the adventure and the strength it brings with it.
   - good Affirmations: Repeat daily affirmations to reinforce a good self-image. Statements such as "I am beautiful" and "I am enough" might change your perspective.

2. Mental and Emotional Well-Being: - Mindfulness and Meditation: These activities reduce stress, improve self-awareness, and promote emotional equilibrium, resulting in an inner glow.
   - Therapy and Counselling: Professional assistance can help address any remaining self-esteem issues and build a positive self-image.

3. Purpose and Passion: - Pursue Interests: Participate in activities that provide joy and fulfilment. Passionate interests increase your zest for life and reflect it.

- Volunteer and Give Back: Helping others gives you a sense of purpose and community, which enriches your life and improves your inner beauty.

Outer Glow: Skincare and Self-Care Rituals.

1. Skincare Regimen: - Hydration: Drink plenty of water and use moisturizers appropriate for your skin type. Ceramides and hyaluronic acid are great moisturizers.
   - Sun Protection: Use a broad-spectrum sunscreen to protect your skin from the sun's harm. UV exposure promotes ageing and can cause skin problems.
   - Anti-Age Products: Use products containing retinoids, vitamin C, and peptides to increase collagen production and decrease fine wrinkles.

2. Healthy Nutrition includes a balanced diet. A diet high in antioxidants, vitamins, and minerals improves skin health. Incorporate plenty of fruits, veggies, nuts, and seafood into your meals.
   - Supplies: For skin, hair, and nail health, consider taking omega-3 fatty acids, collagen, or biotin supplements.

3. Exercise and Physical exercise: - Regular Exercise: Physical exercise boosts circulation, delivering oxygen and nutrients to the skin. It also promotes healthy weight and muscle tone.
   - face Exercises: Use face yoga or exercises to tone your facial muscles and increase suppleness.

4. Beauty Treatments: - Facials and Masks: Regular facials and moisturizing masks renew the skin and provide a relaxing experience.
   - Non-Invasive Treatments: Consider microdermabrasion, chemical peels, and laser therapy for skin renewal.

Celebrating Your Unique Style

1. Fashion and Personal Style: - Wardrobe Refresh Update your wardrobe with items that make you feel confident and comfortable. Choose clothing that complements your existing body type.
   - Accessorize: Use scarves, jewelry and purses to show off your personality and add flair to your ensembles.

2. Hair Care: - For healthy hair, use nourishing and strengthening shampoos and conditioners. Regular cuts and treatments can help your hair appear its best.
   - Hair Color: Embrace your natural color, improve it, or try out new tones that make you feel alive.

3. Makeup Tips: - Feature Enhancement Makeup can help to highlight your greatest features. A nice foundation, blush, and mascara may do wonders.
   - The Natural Look: Choose a natural, dewy look that highlights your skin's brightness. Avoid using excessive makeup, since it might settle into fine lines.

Accepting Ageing with Grace

Ageing is a natural process that results in a multitude of experiences and memories. Embracing it with grace includes:

1. Practice gratitude on a daily basis. Cultivate thankfulness for your body's journey. Recognize the strength and resilience it has demonstrated over time.

2. Legacy and Storytelling: - Share Your Story: Reflect on your life's path and share your experiences with others. Your experiences are invaluable and encouraging.
   • Family and Community: Engage with younger generations, handing down knowledge and building relationships.

Conclusion: Radiance comes from inside

Beauty beyond age is more than just physical looks; it is about exuding confidence, joy, and sincerity. At any age, you may embrace your brightness by cultivating both your inner and exterior selves. Celebrate the unique beauty that comes with age, honor your path, and keep shining brightly, knowing that true beauty comes from within.

NOTE

CHAPTER 10:
CONFIDENCE REDEFINED: THRIVING IN YOUR NEW CHAPTER

Chapter 10: Confidence Redefined: Thriving in Your Next Chapter

As you approach the post-menopausal stage, reframing confidence is critical to prospering in this new chapter of life. Confidence is more than just self-assurance; it's about accepting who you are, enjoying your accomplishments, and stepping into your power with grace and resolve. This chapter looks at ways to build and redefine confidence, allowing you to live fully and truthfully.

Embracing Change and Growth

Menopause is a huge adjustment, but it also presents a unique chance for personal development and reinvention. Embracing this transformation can result in increased confidence and a better understanding of yourself.

1. Accept physical changes with self-compassion. Recognize the natural changes and enjoy the adventure your body has taken.
   - Positive Body Image: Focus on your body's abilities rather than its appearance. Celebrate your inner strength, resilience, and the experiences that have shaped you.

2. Emotional Resilience: - **Mindfulness and Meditation**: Regular mindfulness activities can help you stay grounded, reduce anxiety, and improve emotional balance.
   - Therapeutic Support: Seek professional help if necessary to handle emotional difficulties and build resilience.

Developing Self-Confidence

Recognizing your worth, setting realistic goals, and enjoying your accomplishments are all steps towards developing self-confidence. Here are some techniques to help you build and retain confidence:

1. Self-Reflection: - Identify Strengths: Evaluate your strengths and accomplishments. Write them down and refer to them on a regular basis.

   - Set goals: Set short- and long-term goals that are consistent with your values and interests. Achieving these goals can increase your self-esteem and sense of purpose.

2. Continuous Learning: - Embrace New Skills: Commit to lifetime learning. Take up new hobbies, enroll in classes, or explore activities that will keep your mind active and happy.

   - Stay curious: Develop a curious mindset. Ask inquiries, seek out new experiences, and be open to change.

3. Self-Care: - Physical Activity: Regular exercise enhances physical health, mood, and confidence. Select activities that you enjoy and that make you feel powerful and capable.

   - A Healthy Lifestyle: To preserve general health, prioritize a well-balanced diet, proper sleep, and stress-management skills.

Empowering Yourself with Connections
Building and sustaining relationships can have a major impact on your confidence. Surround yourself with encouraging people who encourage and inspire you.
1. Social Networks: - Stay Connected: Maintain relationships with loved ones. Engage in social activities that promote connection and belonging.

   - Seek Support: Join support groups or online forums to share your experiences and learn from others going through similar adjustments.

2. Mentorship and Role Models: - Find Mentors: Identify mentors who can offer guidance, support, and encouragement as you embark on this new chapter.

   - Become a Role Model: Share your experiences and knowledge with others. Mentoring can enhance your confidence and provide a sense of accomplishment.

Thrive in Your Career and Passions

Post menopause might be an opportunity to reconsider your career and ambitions. Whether you want to stay in your current industry, switch careers, or follow personal hobbies, success in this area is critical for sustaining confidence.

1. Career Development: - Skills Enhancement: Constantly improve your skills and knowledge. Attend workshops, get certified, and keep current in your field.
   - Networking: Establish a professional network. Attend industry events, join professional associations, and network with colleagues.

2. Pursuing Passions: - Creative Outlets: Enjoy creative pursuits like painting, writing, gardening, or music.
   - Volunteering: Contribute to the community through voluntary labor. Contributing to causes that you care about can give you a sense of purpose and boost your self-esteem.

Developing a Positive Mindset

A positive outlook is the cornerstone of confidence. How you see difficulties and opportunities has a huge impact on your confidence.

1. Positive Thinking: - Affirmations: Reinforce confidence with positive affirmations. Statements like "I am capable" and "I trust my abilities" can help you change your mind.
   - appreciation Practice: Cultivate appreciation by consistently noticing the positive aspects in your life. This activity can boost happiness and confidence.

2. To overcome negative self-talk, identify and confront limiting ideas that hinder confidence. Replace them with empowering thoughts.

   - Surround Yourself with Positivity: Consume positive, uplifting content, such as books, podcasts, and media, to inspire and motivate yourself.

Redefining Success

In this new chapter, redefine your definition of success. Success is not a one-size fits all concept; rather, it is a very personal and developing journey.

1. To achieve personal fulfilment, match your pursuits with your basic values and passions. This congruence promotes a sense of authenticity and fulfilment.

   - appreciate Milestones: Recognize and appreciate your accomplishments, no matter how minor. Each stride forward demonstrates your resilience and improvement.

2. Maintain a balanced life by integrating work and personal life. Integrate work, personal interests, family, and self-care in a way that seems natural.

   - Flexibility and Adaptability: Maintain flexibility and adaptability to change. Accept new opportunities and be prepared to pivot as necessary.

Conclusion: Stepping into Your Power

Confidence redefined entails accepting all of who you are—your experiences, strengths, and goals. You can succeed in this new chapter by focusing on personal development, fostering relationships, following your passions, and cultivating a positive mindset. Step into your power with confidence, knowing that your journey is unique and worthwhile. Accept this moment as an opportunity to rediscover yourself, redefine success, and live fully and truly.

NOTE

CONCLUSION

Conclusion: Accepting the New Body Menopause
As we near the end of our trip through "Menopause Revival Power," it's time to reflect on the lessons learned and embrace this new chapter of life with confidence, vigor, and joy. Menopause is a transitional moment that marks the end of one stage and the start of another, full of opportunity for growth, self-discovery, and newfound purpose.

Accepting Change with Grace

Menopause causes profound changes to your body, mind, and emotions. It's a period of transition that can be both difficult and rewarding. Understanding and accepting these changes allows you to approach menopause with a good attitude. Acceptance marks the first step towards empowerment. Acknowledge your body's physical shifts, emotional fluctuations, and new rhythms. Accept them as natural steps in your life's path.

Holistic Health and Well-Being

Throughout this book, we've emphasized the value of a comprehensive approach to health. Menopause is more than just treating symptoms; it is about nurturing your full being. Holistic health refers to physical, mental, and emotional well-being.

1. Physical Health: Prioritize nutrition, exercise, and preventative care. A well-balanced diet, frequent physical activity, and routine medical check-ups are essential for preserving overall health and vigor.
2. Mental Health: Practice mindfulness, seek professional help when needed, and remain mentally engaged. Mental health is essential in navigating the emotional landscape of menopause.
3. Emotional Health*: Strengthen your social ties, practice self-compassion, and embrace emotional resilience. Emotional health is essential for feeling connected, loved, and supported.

Redefining Beauty and Confidence.

Menopause allows you to redefine beauty and confidence on your own terms. Beauty is timeless and multifaceted, encompassing not just physical appearance but also inner power, knowledge, and honesty. Confidence redefined means accepting your unique shine and stepping into your power.

1. Inner Radiance: Practice self-love, follow passions, and participate in things that offer you joy and fulfilment. Your inner glow comes from living a life that is consistent with your values and passions.
2. Outer Glow: Invest on skincare, clothes, and self-care routines that make you feel lively and confident. Accept your inherent beauty and showcase your unique flair.

Thriving In The Third Age

The post-menopausal years, also known as the "third age," can be among the most rewarding of your life. This period provides an opportunity to find yourself, pursue long-held aspirations, and make a meaningful contribution to your community. Thriving in this stage includes:

1. Purpose and Passion: Participate in things that spark your passions and give you a sense of purpose. Discover what makes you feel alive, whether through creative endeavors, volunteering, or lifelong study.
2. Personal Growth: Continue to learn, develop, and change. Accept new challenges, make new goals, and stay curious about the world around you.
3. Community and Connection: Build strong bonds with family, friends, and like-minded people. Strong social networks offer support, excitement, and a sense of belonging.

Practical Strategies for a Balanced Lifestyle

Throughout this book, we have presented practical solutions for dealing with the various facets of menopause. These strategies are designed to help you manage this shift smoothly and gracefully:

1. Stress Management: Add mindfulness, meditation, and relaxation practices to your everyday routine. Effective stress management is essential for maintaining emotional balance.
2. nutritious Lifestyle Choices: Prioritize a nutritious diet, regular exercise, and enough sleep. These lifestyle choices are the cornerstone of your well-being.
3. Preventive Health Care: Stay on top of your health by scheduling frequent screenings and check-ups. Early detection and prevention are critical to long-term health.

Accepting Your Unique Journey

Each woman's menopausal experience is unique. There is no one-size-fits-all solution, and it is critical to determine what works best for you. Listen to your body, trust your instincts, and seek knowledge and help that is specific to your needs. View this trip as an opportunity for self-discovery and empowerment.

The Power of Self-Compassion

Finally, face the new chapter with self-compassion. Be gentle with yourself while you experience the ups and downs of menopause. Celebrate your accomplishments, learn from your setbacks, and respect your journey. Self-compassion is the foundation of a satisfying and fulfilled existence.

Looking Forward

As you move forward, keep the knowledge and ideas you received from this book with you. Allow them to guide you through the new body menopause with confidence and grace. This is a time to honor your courage, wisdom, and the wonderful journey that has led you to this point.

Remember that menopause is a new beginning—an opportunity to redefine yourself, your health, your beauty, and your confidence. Accept this new chapter with an open heart and a strong spirit, knowing that the best is still to come. Thank you for going on this adventure with me. Here's to thriving, flourishing, and living your best life during menopause.

NOTE

APPENDIX

Appendix: Resources for Thriving in Menopause

As you continue your journey through menopause and beyond, having access to reliable resources can provide invaluable support and guidance. This appendix offers a curated list of books, websites, support groups, and professional organizations that can help you navigate this transformative stage of life with confidence and ease.

Recommended Reading

1. Books on Menopause and Women's Health:
   - "The Wisdom of Menopause" by Dr. Christiane Northrup: A comprehensive guide that explores the physical and emotional changes of menopause, offering practical advice and insights.
   - "Menopause Matters: Your Guide to a Long and Healthy Life" by Dr. Julia Schram Edelman: This book provides clear and concise information on managing menopause symptoms and maintaining health.
   - "The Hormone Cure" by Dr. Sara Gottfried: Focuses on balancing hormones naturally through diet, exercise, and lifestyle changes.
   - "What Your Doctor May Not Tell You About Menopause" by Dr. John R. Lee and Virginia Hopkins: Offers a perspective on natural hormone replacement therapy and holistic approaches to menopause.

2. Books on Mindfulness and Well-Being:
   - "The Miracle of Mindfulness" by Thich Nhat Han: A foundational book on mindfulness practices that can help manage stress and enhance well-being.
   - **"Radical Acceptance" by Tara Brach**: Explores the power of self-compassion and mindfulness in overcoming life's challenges.

Online Resources

1. Informative Websites:
   - North American Menopause Society (NAMS)
   Offers comprehensive information on menopause, including symptoms, treatment options, and latest research.
   - National Institute on Aging (NIA)   Provides resources on aging, health, and menopause, including expert-reviewed articles and guides.
   - Menopause Matters   A website dedicated to providing independent advice and information on menopause, symptoms, and treatments.

2. Supportive Communities:
   - Red Hot Mamas
   An educational organization that offers support groups, forums, and resources for women experiencing menopause.
   - Menopause Chicks:
   An online community and resource hub where women can share experiences and find expert advice on menopause and midlife health.

Support Groups and Networks

1. Local and Online Support Groups:
   - Meetup:
   Search for menopause support groups in your area or join virtual meetups to connect with other women going through similar experiences.
   - Facebook Groups: Search for menopause-related groups on Facebook to find communities where you can share, learn, and receive support.

2. Professional Organizations:
   - American Menopause Foundation:
   Provides resources and support for women navigating menopause,
including information on hormone therapy and health management.
   - International Menopause Society (IMS)
   A global organization offering educational materials, research updates,
and support for healthcare professionals and women experiencing
menopause.

Holistic and Alternative Health Resources

1. Holistic Health Practitioners:
   - National Association for Holistic Aromatherapy (NAHA):
   Find certified aromatherapists who can guide you in using essential oils
for menopause symptom relief.
   - American Association of Naturopathic Physicians (AANP):
www.naturopathic.org
   Locate licensed naturopathic doctors who specialize in women's health
and menopause.

2. Alternative Medicine:
   - Acupuncture: Consider finding a licensed acupuncturist to explore how
acupuncture can help alleviate menopause symptoms.
   - Yoga and Meditation Centers: Search for local yoga studios or
meditation centers offering classes specifically designed for menopause and
midlife women.

thanks for reading

NOTE

NOTE

NOTE

NOTE

NOTE